JUICING AND SMOOTHIES FOR PROSTATE CANCER REVERSAL

60 quick and easy anti cancer fruit blends and juices to manage, prevent and recover from Adenocarcinoma of the prostate

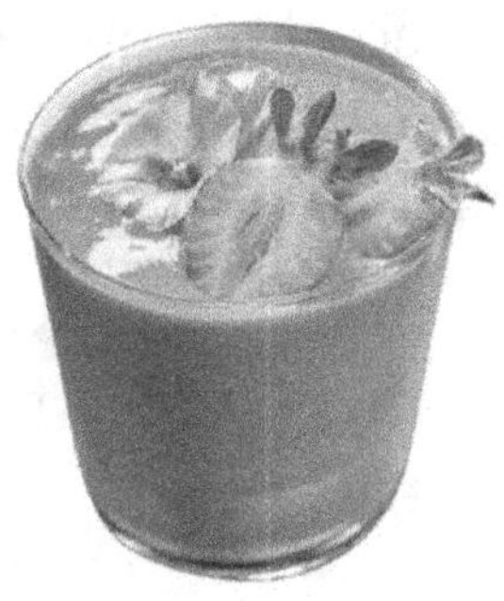

Dr. Malvin Harison

TABLE OF CONTENT

Introduction 3

    Overview 5

    Causes of Prostate Cancer 8

Chapter 1: Juicing For Prostate Cancer Reversal 11

    General instructions for all the juices 11

    1. Green Vitality Boost 11

    2. Berry Bliss Elixir 12

    3. Turmeric Tango Tonic 12

    4. Citrus Cleanse Splash 13

    5. Carrot-Apple Revitalizer 13

    6. Cranberry Prostate Protector 14

    7. Pineapple-Turmeric Zinger 14

    8. Spinach-Berry Bliss..................................15

    9. Gingered Watermelon Wonder 16

    10. Broccoli-Pear Powerhouse 16

    11. Tomato-Basil Prostate Tonic....................17

    12. Mango-Turmeric Fusion 17

    13. Avocado-Kale Elixir.................................18

    14. Cherry-Almond Bliss 18

    15. Cucumber-Mint Hydration Splash 19

    16. Raspberry-Beet Radiance........................19

    17. Papaya-Coconut Refresher 20

    18. Spinach-Avocado Detoxifier.....................20

    19. Apricot-Ginger Euphoria 21

    20. Kale-Pineapple Reviver 21

    21. Blueberry-Coconut Bliss 22

    22. Cantaloupe-Carrot Crush.........................22

23. Strawberry-Basil Refresher 23

24. Minty Watercress Detox 23

25. Plum-Grape Antioxidant Boost 24

26. Beetroot-Orange Energizer 24

27. Cherry-Almond Protein Refuel 25

28. Peach-Ginger Cooler 25

29. Celery-Apple Hydration Splash 26

30. Pomegranate-Kale Vitality Burst 26

Chapter 2: Smoothies Recipes for Prostate cancer reversal 28

1. Berry-Protein Powerhouse 28

2. Spinach-Pineapple Refresher 29

3. Turmeric-Berry Boost 29

4. Cranberry-Walnut Warrior 30

5. Papaya-Coconut Bliss 30

6. Blueberry-Almond Energy Elixir 31

7. Watermelon-Mint Detox Splash 32

8. Protein-Packed Peanut Butter Delight 32

9. Avocado-Berry Bliss 33

10. Cucumber-Parsley Detox Delight 33

11. Cherry-Almond Protein Refuel 34

12. Mango-Turmeric Tropical Delight 35

13. Kiwi-Strawberry Sensation 35

14. Beetroot-Berry Antioxidant Blast 36

15. Peach-Oat Power Smoothie 36

16. Orange-Mango Immunity Boost 37

17. Blueberry-Coconut Dream 38

18. Chia-Berry Omega-3 Delight 38

19. Raspberry-Coconut Hydration Refresher .. 39

20. Mango-Coconut Paradise 39

21. Pomegranate-Protein Punch.....................40

22. Strawberry-Banana Oatmeal Delight 40

23. Watermelon-Cucumber Cool Down 41

24. Almond-Cherry Recovery Smoothie 42

25. Cantaloupe-Carrot Glow 42

26. Blueberry-Beet Antioxidant Boost 43

27. Peach-Ginger Hydration Elixir...................43

28. Raspberry-Almond Protein Smoothie 44

29. Strawberry-Banana Oatmeal Delight 45

30. Apricot-Almond Refuel 45

Chapter 3: BONUS 47

21 exercises for prostate cancer patients 47

Conclusion 50

Introduction

Embark on a tantalizing journey to reverse prostate cancer through the vibrant world of juicing and smoothies. Brace yourself for a mouthwatering adventure as we explore the delicious synergy of nature's bounty and potent nutrients.

These concoctions are not just tasty; they're your allies in the fight for prostate health. Let's sip our way to vitality, one flavorful blend at a time. Welcome to the ultimate fusion of taste and wellness.

Overview

Prostate cancer is a type of cancer that occurs in the prostate, a small walnut-shaped gland that produces seminal fluid in men. It is one of the most common cancers among men, typically developing slowly and often without symptoms in its early stages. **Here's an overview:**

1. Incidence: Prostate Cancer, second most common cancer in men on earth, is a prevalent cancer, especially in older men.

2. Age and Risk: The risk of prostate cancer increases with age, and it is more commonly diagnosed in men over the age of 50. The majority of cases are found in men over 65.

3. Symptoms: Early-stage prostate cancer often presents with no symptoms. As the cancer progresses, symptoms may include difficulty urinating, frequent urination (especially at night), blood in the urine or semen, pain or discomfort in the pelvic area, and erectile dysfunction.

4. Diagnosis: Prostate cancer is typically detected through a combination of a digital rectal examination (DRE) and a blood test measuring prostate-specific antigen (PSA) levels. Biopsy may be performed for confirmation.

5. Grading and Staging: The cancer is graded based on the Gleason score, which evaluates the aggressiveness of the cancer cells.

6. Treatment Options: Treatment options depend on the stage and aggressiveness of the cancer. Common approaches include active surveillance, surgery (prostatectomy), radiation therapy, hormone therapy, chemotherapy, and immunotherapy.

7. Survival Rates: Prostate cancer often has a high survival rate, especially when detected and treated early. The prognosis varies based on factors such as the stage, grade, and overall health of the individual.

8. Risk Factors: Risk factors include age, family history, genetic factors, race (African-American men have a higher risk), and certain lifestyle factors.

9. Prevention: While the exact cause is unknown, adopting a healthy lifestyle, including a balanced diet rich in fruits and vegetables, regular exercise, and avoiding tobacco, may contribute to lowering the risk.

Causes of Prostate Cancer

The exact causes of prostate cancer are not fully understood, but several factors are known to contribute to its development. It's often a result of a combination of genetic, environmental, and lifestyle factors.

Here are some key factors associated with the development of prostate cancer:

1. Age: The risk of prostate cancer increases with age, and it is more common in men over the age of 50. It is mostly diagnosed in older men.

2. Family History: Individuals with a family history of prostate cancer, especially in first-degree relatives (father, brother), have a higher risk.

3. Genetic Factors: Certain inherited gene mutations, such as BRCA1 and BRCA2, have been linked to an increased risk of prostate cancer.

4. Race and Ethnicity: African-American men have a higher incidence of prostate cancer compared to men of other racial and ethnic groups. The cause for these disparities are not well understood.

5. Geography: Prostate cancer rates vary geographically, with higher incidence rates in North America, Europe, and Australia.

6. Hormonal Factors: Androgens, particularly testosterone, play a role in the development and growth of prostate cancer. Men with higher levels of androgens may be at an increased risk.

7. Dietary Factors: Diets high in red and processed meats and low in fruits and vegetables may be associated with an increased risk of prostate cancer.

8. Obesity: There is evidence suggesting that obesity may be linked to a higher risk of aggressive prostate cancer.

9.   Inflammation: Chronic inflammation of the prostate (prostatitis) may be associated with an increased risk of prostate cancer.

10. Occupational Exposures: Some studies have explored potential links between certain occupational exposures (e.g., to cadmium, pesticides) and an elevated risk of prostate cancer.

Chapter 1: Juicing For Prostate Cancer Reversal

General instructions for all the juices

1. Rinse the vegetables and fruits very well.

2. Cut them into manageable pieces for your juicer.

3. Juice all the ingredients, ensuring a well-blended mixture.

4. Pour the juice into a glass and stir gently.

5. Consume immediately for maximum freshness and nutritional benefit.

1. Green Vitality Boost

Ingredients

- 2 cups kale
- 1 cucumber
- 1 green apple
- 1 lemon (peeled)
- 1-inch ginger (peeled)

Serving Size: 1-2 servings

Nutritional Value: High in antioxidants, vitamins A and C.
Cooking Time: 10 minutes

2. Berry Bliss Elixir

Ingredients
- 1 cup blueberries
- 1 cup strawberries
- 1/2 cup pomegranate seeds
- 1 beetroot (peeled)
- 1 tablespoon flax seeds

Serving Size: 2 servings
Nutritional Value: Rich in fiber, vitamin C, and antioxidants.
Cooking Time: 8 minutes

3. Turmeric Tango Tonic

Ingredients
- 2 carrots
- 1 orange (peeled)
- 1/2 inch turmeric root (or 1 tsp turmeric powder)
- 1/2 lemon (peeled)
- 1 tablespoon chia seeds

Serving Size: 1-2 servings
Nutritional Value: Anti-inflammatory, high in vitamin A and antioxidants.
Cooking Time: 7 minutes

4. Citrus Cleanse Splash

Ingredients
- 2 grapefruits (peeled)
- 1 lime (peeled)
- 1 cup pineapple chunks
- 1 cucumber
- 1 tablespoon mint leaves

Serving Size: 2 servings
Nutritional Value: Detoxifying, rich in vitamin C and hydrating.
Cooking Time: 5 minutes

5. Carrot-Apple Revitalizer

Ingredients
- 3 carrots
- 2 apples
- 1/2 inch ginger (peeled)
- 1 tablespoon hemp seeds

Serving Size: 1-2 servings
Nutritional Value: High in beta-carotene, vitamin K, and omega-3 fatty acids.
Cooking Time: 6 minutes

6. Cranberry Prostate Protector

Ingredients
- 1 cup cranberries
- 1 pear
- 1/2 cucumber
- 1 tablespoon pumpkin seeds

Serving Size: 2 servings
Nutritional Value: Antioxidant-rich, supports urinary health.
Cooking Time: 7 minutes

7. Pineapple-Turmeric Zinger

Ingredients
- 1 cup pineapple chunks
- 1/2 inch turmeric root (or 1 tsp turmeric powder)
- 1 orange (peeled)
- 1 carrot

Serving Size: 1-2 servings
Nutritional Value: Anti-inflammatory, high in vitamin C and manganese.
Cooking Time: 6 minutes

8. Spinach-Berry Bliss

Ingredients
   - 2 cups spinach
   - 1 cup mixed berries (strawberries, raspberries, blueberries)
   - 1 banana
   - 1 tablespoon chia seeds
Serving Size: 2 servings
Nutritional Value: Rich in iron, vitamin C, and antioxidants.
Cooking Time: 5 minutes

9. Gingered Watermelon Wonder

Ingredients

- 2 cups watermelon chunks
- 1/2 inch ginger (peeled)
- 1 lime (peeled)
- 1 cucumber

Serving Size: 1-2 servings
Nutritional Value: Hydrating, supports immune function.
Cooking Time: 4 minutes

10. Broccoli-Pear Powerhouse

Ingredients

- 1 cup broccoli florets
- 1 pear
- 1 celery stalk
- 1/2 lemon (peeled)

Serving Size: 2 servings
Nutritional Value: High in fiber, vitamin C, and potassium.
Cooking Time: 8 minutes

11. Tomato-Basil Prostate Tonic

Ingredients
- 4 tomatoes
- Handful of fresh basil leaves
- 1 bell pepper (any color)
- 1 celery stalk

Serving Size: 2 servings
Nutritional Value: Rich in lycopene, vitamin C, and potassium.
Cooking Time: 8 minutes

12. Mango-Turmeric Fusion

Ingredients
- 2 cups mango chunks
- 1/2 inch turmeric root (or 1 tsp turmeric powder)
- 1 orange (peeled)
- 1 carrot

Serving Size: 1-2 servings
Nutritional Value: Anti-inflammatory, high in vitamin A and antioxidants.
Cooking Time: 6 minutes

13. Avocado-Kale Elixir

Ingredients
- 1 avocado
- 2 cups kale
- 1 green apple
- 1 lemon (peeled)

Serving Size: 2 servings
Nutritional Value: Packed with healthy fats, vitamins A and C.
Cooking Time: 7 minutes

14. Cherry-Almond Bliss

Ingredients
- 1 cup cherries (pitted)
- 1 banana
- 1 cup almond milk
- 1 tablespoon almond butter

Serving Size: 2 servings
Nutritional Value: Rich in antioxidants, potassium, and healthy fats.
Cooking Time: 5 minutes

15.   Cucumber-Mint   Hydration Splash

Ingredients
- 2 cucumbers
- Handful of fresh mint leaves
- 1 lime (peeled)
- 1/2 cup coconut water

Serving Size: 1-2 servings
Nutritional   Value: Hydrating, supports digestion.
Cooking Time: 5 minutes

16. Raspberry-Beet Radiance

Ingredients
- 1 cup raspberries
- 1 beetroot (peeled)
- 1 orange (peeled)
- 1 tablespoon flax seeds

Serving Size: 2 servings
Nutritional Value: High in fiber, vitamin C, and antioxidants.
Cooking Time: 7 minutes

17. Papaya-Coconut Refresher

Ingredients
- 2 cups papaya chunks
- 1/2 cup coconut milk
- 1 banana
- 1 tablespoon chia seeds

Serving Size: 1-2 servings
Nutritional Value: Rich in papain, vitamin C, and healthy fats.
Cooking Time: 6 minutes

18. Spinach-Avocado Detoxifier

Ingredients
- 2 cups spinach
- 1 avocado
- 1 cucumber
- 1/2 lemon (peeled)

Serving Size: 2 servings
Nutritional Value: Detoxifying, high in vitamins A and K.
Cooking Time: 7 minutes

19. Apricot-Ginger Euphoria

Ingredients

- 1 cup apricots (pitted)
- 1/2 inch ginger (peeled)
- 1 apple
- 1 tablespoon hemp seeds

Serving Size: 1-2 servings

Nutritional Value: Anti-inflammatory, high in vitamin C and omega-3 fatty acids.

Cooking Time: 6 minutes

20. Kale-Pineapple Reviver

Ingredients

- 2 cups kale
- 1 cup pineapple chunks
- 1 banana
- 1 tablespoon pumpkin seeds

Serving Size: 2 servings.

Nutritional Value: Rich in fiber, vitamin C, and potassium.

Cooking Time: 5 minutes

21. Blueberry-Coconut Bliss

Ingredients
- 1 cup blueberries
- 1/2 cup coconut water
- 1 banana
- Handful of spinach

Serving Size: 2 servings
Nutritional Value: Rich in antioxidants, potassium, and electrolytes.
Cooking Time: 5 minutes

22. Cantaloupe-Carrot Crush

Ingredients
- 2 cups cantaloupe chunks
- 2 carrots
- 1 orange (peeled)
- 1/2 inch ginger (peeled)

Serving Size: 1-2 servings
Nutritional Value: High in vitamin A, vitamin C, and beta-carotene.
Cooking Time: 6 minutes

23. Strawberry-Basil Refresher

Ingredients
- 1 cup strawberries
- Handful of fresh basil leaves
- 1 apple
- 1/2 lemon (peeled)

Serving Size: 2 servings
Nutritional Value: Antioxidant-rich, with a burst of vitamin C.
Cooking Time: 7 minutes

24. Minty Watercress Detox

Ingredients
- 2 cups watercress
- Handful of fresh mint leaves
- 1 cucumber
- 1 green apple

Serving Size: 1-2 servings
Nutritional Value: Detoxifying, high in vitamin K and antioxidants.
Cooking Time: 8 minutes

25. Plum-Grape Antioxidant Boost

Ingredients
- 1 cup red grapes
- 2 plums (pitted)
- 1/2 cucumber
- 1 tablespoon flax seeds

Serving Size: 2 servings
Nutritional Value: Rich in antioxidants, fiber, and vitamin K.
Cooking Time: 7 minutes

26. Beetroot-Orange Energizer

Ingredients
- 1 beetroot (peeled)
- 2 oranges (peeled)
- 1 carrot
- 1 tablespoon chia seeds

Serving Size: 1-2 servings
Nutritional Value: High in iron, vitamin C, and omega-3 fatty acids.
Cooking Time: 8 minutes

27. Cherry-Almond Protein Refuel

Ingredients
- 1 cup cherries (pitted)
- 1/2 cup almond milk
- 1 banana
- 1 scoop plant-based protein powder

Serving Size: 2 servings
Nutritional Value: Protein-packed, rich in antioxidants.
Cooking Time: 5 minutes

28. Peach-Ginger Cooler

Ingredients
- 2 peaches (pitted)
- 1/2 inch ginger (peeled)
- 1 pear
- 1 tablespoon hemp seed

Serving Size: 1-2 servings
Nutritional Value: Anti-inflammatory, high in vitamin C and omega-3 fatty acids.
Cooking Time: 6 minutes

29. Celery-Apple Hydration Splash

Ingredients
- 3 celery stalks
- 2 apples
- 1 cucumber
- 1/2 lemon (peeled)

Serving Size: 2 servings
Nutritional Value: Hydrating, supports digestion.
Cooking Time: 5 minutes

30. Pomegranate-Kale Vitality Burst

Ingredients
- 1 cup pomegranate seeds
- 2 cups kale
- 1 green apple
- 1/2 lime (peeled)

Serving Size: 1-2 servings
Nutritional Value: Rich in antioxidants, vitamins A and K.
Cooking Time: 7 minutes

Chapter 2: Smoothies Recipes for Prostate cancer reversal

Here are 30 smoothie recipes tailored for potential support in prostate health.

1. Berry-Protein Powerhouse

Ingredients
- 1 cup mixed berries
- 1 banana
- 1 scoop plant-based protein powder
- 1 cup almond milk

Instructions
- Blend all ingredients until smooth.

Serving Size: 2 servings

Nutritional Value: Protein-packed, rich in antioxidants.

Preparation Time: 5 minutes

2. Spinach-Pineapple Refresher

Ingredients

- 2 cups spinach
- 1 cup pineapple chunks
- 1/2 cucumber
- 1/2 lime (peeled)

Instructions

- Blend ingredients until well combined.

Serving Size: 1-2 servings

Nutritional Value: High in vitamins A and C, hydrating.

Preparation Time: 4 minutes

3. Turmeric-Berry Boost

Ingredients

- 1 cup mixed berries
- 1/2 teaspoon turmeric powder
- 1 banana
- 1 cup coconut water

Instructions

- Blend until smooth.

Serving Size: 1-2 servings

Nutritional Value: Anti-inflammatory, rich in antioxidants.

Preparation Time: 5 minutes

4. Cranberry-Walnut Warrior

Ingredients
- 1 cup cranberries
- 1/4 cup walnuts
- 1 banana
- 1 cup Greek yogurt

Instructions
- Blend ingredients until creamy.

Serving Size: 2 servings

Nutritional Value: Omega-3 fatty acids, protein.

Preparation Time: 5 minutes

5. Papaya-Coconut Bliss

Ingredients
- 2 cups papaya chunks
- 1/2 cup coconut milk
- 1 banana
- 1 tablespoon chia seeds

Instructions
- Blend until well combined.

Serving Size: 1-2 servings

Nutritional Value: Healthy fats, digestive support.
Preparation Time: 6 minutes

6. Blueberry-Almond Energy Elixir

Ingredients
- 1 cup blueberries
- 1/4 cup almonds (soaked)
- 1 banana
- 1 cup almond milk

Instructions
- Blend until smooth and creamy.

Serving Size: 2 servings
Nutritional Value: Protein, antioxidants, vitamin E.
Preparation Time: 6 minutes

7. Watermelon-Mint Detox Splash

Ingredients
- 2 cups watermelon chunks
- Handful of fresh mint leaves
- 1/2 cucumber
- 1/2 lemon (peeled)

Instructions
- Blend until refreshing.

Serving Size: 1-2 servings
Nutritional Value: Hydration, digestive support.
Preparation Time: 5 minutes

8. Protein-Packed Peanut Butter Delight

Ingredients
- 1 banana
- 2 tablespoons peanut butter
- 1 cup Greek yogurt
- 1 tablespoon chia seeds

Instructions
- Blend until creamy.

Serving Size: 2 servings

Nutritional Value: Protein, potassium.
Preparation Time: 5 minutes

9. Avocado-Berry Bliss

Ingredients
- 1/2 avocado
- 1 cup mixed berries
- 1 banana
- 1 cup coconut water

Instructions
- Blend until smooth.

Serving Size: 1-2 servings
Nutritional Value: Healthy fats, antioxidants.
Preparation Time: 5 minutes

10. Cucumber-Parsley Detox Delight

Ingredients
- 1 cucumber
- Handful of fresh parsley
- 1 green apple
- 1/2 lemon (peeled)

Instructions
- Blend until detoxifying.
Serving Size: 1-2 servings
Nutritional Value: Cleansing, high in vitamins.
Preparation Time: 5 minutes

11. Cherry-Almond Protein Refuel

Ingredient
- 1 cup cherries (pitted)
- 1/2 cup almond milk
- 1 banana
- 1 scoop plant-based protein powder
Instructions
- Blend until protein-packed.
Serving Size: 2 serving
Nutritional Value: Protein, antioxidants.
Preparation Time: 5 minutes

12.   Mango-Turmeric   Tropical Delight

Ingredients
   - 1 cup mango chunks
   - 1/2 inch turmeric root (or 1 tsp turmeric powder)
   - 1 banana
   - 1 cup Greek yogurt

Instructions
   - Blend until tropical goodness.

Serving Size: 2 servings

Nutritional   Value: Anti-inflammatory, vitamin C.

Preparation Time: 6 minutes

13. Kiwi-Strawberry Sensation

Ingredients
   - 2 kiwis (peeled)
   - 1 cup strawberries
   - 1 banana
   - 1/2 lime (peeled)

Instructions
   - Blend until sensational.

Serving Size: 2 servings

Nutritional Value: Vitamin C, antioxidants.
Preparation Time: 6 minutes

14. Beetroot-Berry Antioxidant Blast

Ingredients
- 1 small beetroot (peeled)
- 1 cup mixed berries
- 1 banana
- 1 cup coconut water

Instructions
- Blend until a vibrant blast.

Serving Size: 1-2 servings
Nutritional Value: Antioxidants, electrolytes.
Preparation Time: 7 minutes

15. Peach-Oat Power Smoothie

Ingredients
- 2 peaches (pitted)
- 1/4 cup oats (soaked)
- 1 cup almond milk
- 1 tablespoon chia seeds

Instructions
- Blend until a power-packed smoothie.
Serving Size: 2 servings
Nutritional Value: High in fiber, vitamins.
Preparation Time: 5 minutes

16. Orange-Mango Immunity Boost

Ingredients
- 2 oranges (peeled)
- 1 cup mango chunks
- 1/2 inch ginger (peeled)
- 1 tablespoon flax seeds

Instructions
- Blend for an immunity boost.
Serving Size: 1-2 servings
Nutritional Value: Vitamin C, antioxidants.
Preparation Time: 7 minutes

17. Blueberry-Coconut Dream

Ingredients
- 1 cup blueberries
- 1/2 cup coconut water
- 1 banana
- Handful of spinach

Instructions
- Blend until a dreamy concoction.

Serving Size: 2 servings

Nutritional Value: Antioxidants, electrolytes.

Preparation Time: 5 minutes

18. Chia-Berry Omega-3 Delight

Ingredients
- 1 cup mixed berries
- 2 tablespoons chia seeds
- 1 banana
- 1 cup Greek yogurt

Instructions
- Blend for an omega-3 delight.

Serving Size: 2 servings

Nutritional Value: Protein, omega-3 fatty acids.

Preparation Time: 5 minutes

19. Raspberry-Coconut Hydration Refresher

Ingredients
- 1 cup raspberries
- 1/2 cup coconut milk
- 1 banana
- 1 tablespoon chia seeds

Instructions
- Blend until a hydrating refresher.

Serving Size: 2 servings

Nutritional Value: Hydration, antioxidants.

Preparation Time: 5 minutes

20. Mango-Coconut Paradise

Ingredients
- 1 cup mango chunks
- 1/2 cup coconut milk
- 1 banana
- 1 tablespoon chia seeds

Instructions
- Blend for a tropical paradise.

Serving Size: 1-2 servings
Nutritional Value: Healthy fats, vitamins.
Preparation Time: 5 minutes

21. Pomegranate-Protein Punch

Ingredients
- 1 cup pomegranate seeds
- 1/2 cup cottage cheese
- 1 banana
- 1 tablespoon hemp seeds

Instructions
- Blend for a protein punch.

Serving Size: 2 servings
Nutritional Value: Protein, antioxidants.
Preparation Time: 6 minutes

22. Strawberry-Banana Oatmeal Delight

Ingredients
- 1 cup strawberries
- 2 bananas
- 1/4 cup oats (soaked)

- 1 cup almond milk

Instructions

- Blend for an oatmeal delight.

Serving Size: 2 servings

Nutritional Value: High in fiber, potassium.

Preparation Time: 7 minutes

23. Watermelon-Cucumber Cool Down

Ingredients

- 2 cups watermelon chunks
- 1 cucumber
- 1/2 lime (peeled)
- Handful of mint leaves

Instructions

- Blend for a refreshing cool down.

Serving Size: 1-2 servings

Nutritional Value: Hydration, digestive support.

Preparation Time: 6 minutes

24. Almond-Cherry Recovery Smoothie

Ingredients:
- 1/4 cup almonds (soaked)
- 1 cup cherries (pitted)
- 1 cup almond milk
- 1 tablespoon almond butter

Instructions
- Blend for a recovery smoothie.

Serving Size: 2 servings

Nutritional Value: Protein, antioxidants.

Preparation Time: 5 minutes

25. Cantaloupe-Carrot Glow

Ingredients
- 2 cups cantaloupe chunks
- 2 carrots
- 1 orange (peeled)
- 1/2 inch ginger (peeled)

Instructions
- Blend for a glowing smoothie.

Serving Size: 1-2 servings

Nutritional Value: High in vitamins A and C, beta-carotene.
Preparation Time: 6 minutes

26.   Blueberry-Beet Antioxidant Boost

Ingredients
- 1 cup blueberries
- 1 small beetroot (peeled)
- 1 banana
- 1/2 cup Greek yogurt

Instructions
- Blend for a refreshing cool down.
Serving Size: 2 servings
Nutritional Value: Rich in antioxidants, protein and fiber.
Preparation Time: 6 minutes

27. Peach-Ginger Hydration Elixir

Ingredients
- 2 peaches (pitted)
- 1/2 inch ginger (peeled)
- 1 cup coconut water
- 1/2 lime (peeled)

Instructions
- Blend until sensational.
Serving Size: 1-2 servings
Nutritional Value: Hydrating, aids digestion.
Preparation Time: 5 minutes

28. Raspberry-Almond Protein Smoothie

Ingredients
- 1 cup raspberries
- 1/4 cup almonds (soaked)
- 1 cup almond milk
- 1 scoop plant-based protein powder

Instructions
- Blend until a vibrant blast.
Serving Size: 2 servings
Nutritional Value: Protein-packed, high in antioxidants and healthy fats.
Preparation Time: 6 minutes

29. Strawberry-Banana Oatmeal Delight

Ingredients
- 1 cup strawberries
- 2 bananas
- 1/4 cup oats (soaked)
- 1 cup almond milk

Instructions
- Blend until sensational.

Serving Size: 2 servings
Nutritional Value: High in fiber, potassium, and protein.
Preparation Time: 7 minutes

30. Apricot-Almond Refuel

Ingredients
- 1 cup apricots (pitted)
- 1/4 cup almonds (soaked)
- 1 cup Greek yogurt
- 1 tablespoon almond butter

Instructions
- Blend for a refueling smoothie.

Serving Size: 2 servings

Nutritional Value: Protein-packed, high in vitamins A and E.
Preparation Time: 5 minutes

Chapter 3: BONUS

21 exercises for prostate cancer patients

Here are 21 general exercises that are commonly recommended for maintaining overall health, but they should be adapted based on individual circumstances:

1. Walking: Engage in brisk walking for at least 30 minutes a day.

2. Cycling: Ride a stationary or regular bike for cardiovascular health.

3. Swimming: Provides a full-body workout with low impact on joints.

4. Strength Training: Include resistance exercises using weights or resistance bands.

5. Yoga: Incorporate gentle yoga poses for flexibility and relaxation.

6. Pilates: Focus on core strength and flexibility.

7. Tai Chi: A slow, meditative martial art that enhances balance and relaxation.

8. Kegel Exercises: Strengthen pelvic floor muscles to improve urinary control.

9. Aerobic Exercises: Include activities like dancing, jumping jacks, or aerobics classes.

10. Balance Exercises: Improve stability with activities like standing on one leg.

11. Stair Climbing: Use stairs for cardiovascular and lower body exercise.

12. Rowing: Engage in rowing exercises for a full-body workout.

13. Circuit Training: Combine strength and cardio exercises in a circuit.

14. Stretching: Incorporate gentle stretches to maintain flexibility.

15. Breathing Exercises: Practice deep breathing for relaxation and stress reduction.

16. Mediation: Include mindfulness practices for mental well-being.

17. Gardening: Engage in light gardening for both physical and mental health.

18. Resistance Band Exercises: Use bands for gentle resistance training.

19. Bodyweight Exercises: Include push-ups, squats, and lunges for strength.

20. Low-Impact Aerobics: Opt for exercises that are easy on the joints.

21. Functional Movements: Mimic daily activities to improve overall functionality.

NOTE: These exercises should be adapted to individual fitness levels and health conditions. Always seek guidance from your healthcare team to ensure a safe and appropriate exercise routine. Additionally, proper nutrition and a healthy lifestyle are essential components of cancer management, so consult with healthcare professionals for comprehensive advice.

Conclusion

Prioritizing prostate health through nutrition can be a flavorful and enjoyable journey. These juicing and smoothie recipes, rich in antioxidants, vitamins, and nutrients, offer a delicious way to support overall well-being. For those navigating prostate cancer or seeking preventive measures, a holistic approach that includes a nutrient-rich diet, regular exercise, and medical guidance is key.

Embracing a variety of colorful fruits, vegetables, and wholesome ingredients not only contributes to prostate health but also adds vibrancy to daily life.
With a commitment to a balanced lifestyle, these recipes can complement your journey towards a healthier and more vibrant you. Here's to good health and the joy of savoring the nourishing goddess of nature!